KEEP UP WITH YOUR PARENT'S DOCTORS ALL IN ONE

Medical Appointment Log Book

DR. JULIE CRENSHAW

Doctor of Physical Therapy
ABPTS Board Certified Specialist in Geriatrics

Help the Caregiver

ISBN-13: 9781737877639
ISBN-10: 1737877635

Cover design by: 100Covers
Printed in the United States of America

KEEP UP WITH YOUR PARENT'S DOCTORS ALL IN ONE

Medical Appointment Log Book

How to Use This Book

Welcome to the best MD communication book ever!

I designed this book with YOU in mind. In my years working in home health, I have had caregivers express the same overwhelm when it comes to keeping up with doctors:

- Where did I put their contact information?
- Why did I forget to ask that question or write down the answer?
- How am I supposed to remember so many different instructions, tests, procedures, and follow ups?
- What am I supposed to do next?!

This book puts all of this information together in ONE place, so you don't ever have to spend time searching or wandering if you forgot something ever again.

This book is meant to keep a permanent record of the things you need to know, not a scratch list of outdated information. Because of this, you will not find pages for appointment dates or medication lists in this book because these things CHANGE and I don't want you carrying around old or incorrect info.

Organize the MD visit pages however makes the most sense to you. Either chronologically, or designate several pages for each doctor. Use the different sections to suit your needs.

I want you to always have an up-to-date and correct medication list with you, so to access your FREE medication list (that can be edited digitally and then printed!) please go to helpthecaregiver.com/medication-list.

My Message to You

I know it can feel overwhelming to have to take on this caregiver role. You can easily feel like the weight of the world is on your shoulders and you're fighting to keep your head above water!

I created Help the Caregiver to provide resources, education, and support for caregivers so no one ever has to feel like they're doing this alone again.

Top tips for using this log book:

- **Keep it in a central location of the house** for easy access and to write down questions for the MD as soon as you think of them.
- **Take it with you to all appointments!** You will take better notes and can refer to information from other doctors.
- **Transfer important MD visit instructions to MD information page** for that doctor.
- Use my companion **Track Your Parent's Vital Signs** log book to learn more about taking and interpreting vitals signs (including when to call the doctor!).

If you're not already: make sure you're following me on YouTube.com/@helpthecaregiver and please join my FREE Facebook group:
www.facebook.com/groups/caregiversofaginglovedones.

Have feedback or questions? Reach out to me at julie@helpthecaregiver.com I'd love to hear from you!

All my best.
Julie

PATIENT INFORMATION

PATIENT

Name: ______________________ **Phone:** ______________________
DOB: ______________________ **Address:** ______________________
Blood type: ______________________ ______________________

EMERGENCY CONTACT #1

Name: ______________________
Phone: ______________________
Relationship: ______________________

EMERGENCY CONTACT #2

Name: ______________________
Phone: ______________________
Relationship: ______________________

INSURANCE #1

Company: ______________________
Plan name: ______________________
Group #: ______________________
ID #: ______________________
Phone #: ______________________

INSURANCE #2

Company: ______________________
Plan name: ______________________
Group #: ______________________
ID #: ______________________
Phone #: ______________________

PHARMACY #1

Name: ______________________
Phone: ______________________
Fax: ______________________
Address: ______________________
____

PHARMACY #2

Name: ______________________
Phone: ______________________
Fax: ______________________
Address: ______________________
____

OTHER:

____
____
____

MD INFORMATION

MD INFO

Name: ______________________

Specialty: ______________________

Notes: ______________________

OFFICE INFO

Phone: ______________________

Address: ______________________

____

STAFF NAMES

Nurse: ______________________

PA/NP: ______________________

Office staff: ______________________

OFFICE INFO CONTINUED

Hours: ______________________

Directions: ______________________

Notes: ______________________

PATIENT PORTAL LOGIN

Website: ______________________

Login ID: ______________________

Password: ______________________

CONDITIONS MD MANAGES

____

____

____

SPECIAL INSTRUCTIONS FROM MD (WHEN TO CALL, RECOMMENDED VITAL SIGN RANGES, WHEN TO TAKE "AS NEEDED" MEDS, ETC.)

____

____

____

____

____

____

____

____

____

MD INFORMATION

MD INFO

Name: ____________________
Specialty: ____________________
Notes: ____________________

OFFICE INFO

Phone: ____________________
Address: ____________________

STAFF NAMES

Nurse: ____________________
PA/NP: ____________________
Office staff: ____________________

OFFICE INFO CONTINUED

Hours: ____________________
Directions: ____________________
Notes: ____________________

PATIENT PORTAL LOGIN

Website: ____________________
Login ID: ____________________
Password: ____________________

CONDITIONS MD MANAGES

SPECIAL INSTRUCTIONS FROM MD (WHEN TO CALL, RECOMMENDED VITAL SIGN RANGES, WHEN TO TAKE "AS NEEDED" MEDS, ETC.)

MD INFORMATION

MD INFO

Name: ____________________

Specialty: ____________________

Notes: ____________________

OFFICE INFO

Phone: ____________________

Address: ____________________

____

STAFF NAMES

Nurse: ____________________

PA/NP: ____________________

Office staff: ____________________

OFFICE INFO CONTINUED

Hours: ____________________

Directions: ____________________

Notes: ____________________

PATIENT PORTAL LOGIN

Website: ____________________

Login ID: ____________________

Password: ____________________

CONDITIONS MD MANAGES

____

____

____

SPECIAL INSTRUCTIONS FROM MD (WHEN TO CALL, RECOMMENDED VITAL SIGN RANGES, WHEN TO TAKE "AS NEEDED" MEDS, ETC.)

____

____

____

____

____

____

____

____

____

MD INFORMATION

MD INFO

Name: ____________________

Specialty: ____________________

Notes: ____________________

OFFICE INFO

Phone: ____________________

Address: ____________________

____

STAFF NAMES

Nurse: ____________________

PA/NP: ____________________

Office staff: ____________________

OFFICE INFO CONTINUED

Hours: ____________________

Directions: ____________________

Notes: ____________________

PATIENT PORTAL LOGIN

Website: ____________________

Login ID: ____________________

Password: ____________________

CONDITIONS MD MANAGES

____

____

____

SPECIAL INSTRUCTIONS FROM MD (WHEN TO CALL, RECOMMENDED VITAL SIGN RANGES, WHEN TO TAKE "AS NEEDED" MEDS, ETC.)

____

____

____

____

____

____

____

____

____

MD INFORMATION

MD INFO

Name: ______________________

Specialty: ______________________

Notes: ______________________

OFFICE INFO

Phone: ______________________

Address: ______________________

____

STAFF NAMES

Nurse: ______________________

PA/NP: ______________________

Office staff: ______________________

OFFICE INFO CONTINUED

Hours: ______________________

Directions: ______________________

Notes: ______________________

PATIENT PORTAL LOGIN

Website: ______________________

Login ID: ______________________

Password: ______________________

CONDITIONS MD MANAGES

____

____

____

SPECIAL INSTRUCTIONS FROM MD (WHEN TO CALL, RECOMMENDED VITAL SIGN RANGES, WHEN TO TAKE "AS NEEDED" MEDS, ETC.)

____

____

____

____

____

____

____

____

____

MD INFORMATION

MD INFO

Name: ______________________

Specialty: ______________________

Notes: ______________________

OFFICE INFO

Phone: ______________________

Address: ______________________

____

STAFF NAMES

Nurse: ______________________

PA/NP: ______________________

Office staff: ______________________

OFFICE INFO CONTINUED

Hours: ______________________

Directions: ______________________

Notes: ______________________

PATIENT PORTAL LOGIN

Website: ______________________

Login ID: ______________________

Password: ______________________

CONDITIONS MD MANAGES

____

____

____

SPECIAL INSTRUCTIONS FROM MD (WHEN TO CALL, RECOMMENDED VITAL SIGN RANGES, WHEN TO TAKE "AS NEEDED" MEDS, ETC.)

____

____

____

____

____

____

____

____

____

MD INFORMATION

MD INFO

Name: ______________________

Specialty: ______________________

Notes: ______________________

OFFICE INFO

Phone: ______________________

Address: ______________________

____

STAFF NAMES

Nurse: ______________________

PA/NP: ______________________

Office staff: ______________________

OFFICE INFO CONTINUED

Hours: ______________________

Directions: ______________________

Notes: ______________________

PATIENT PORTAL LOGIN

Website: ______________________

Login ID: ______________________

Password: ______________________

CONDITIONS MD MANAGES

____

____

____

SPECIAL INSTRUCTIONS FROM MD (WHEN TO CALL, RECOMMENDED VITAL SIGN RANGES, WHEN TO TAKE "AS NEEDED" MEDS, ETC.)

____

____

____

____

____

____

____

____

____

MD INFORMATION

MD INFO

Name: ____________________

Specialty: ____________________

Notes: ____________________

OFFICE INFO

Phone: ____________________

Address: ____________________

____

STAFF NAMES

Nurse: ____________________

PA/NP: ____________________

Office staff: ____________________

OFFICE INFO CONTINUED

Hours: ____________________

Directions: ____________________

Notes: ____________________

PATIENT PORTAL LOGIN

Website: ____________________

Login ID: ____________________

Password: ____________________

CONDITIONS MD MANAGES

____

____

____

SPECIAL INSTRUCTIONS FROM MD (WHEN TO CALL, RECOMMENDED VITAL SIGN RANGES, WHEN TO TAKE "AS NEEDED" MEDS, ETC.)

____

____

____

____

____

____

____

____

____

MD INFORMATION

MD INFO

Name: ______________________

Specialty: ______________________

Notes: ______________________

OFFICE INFO

Phone: ______________________

Address: ______________________

____

STAFF NAMES

Nurse: ______________________

PA/NP: ______________________

Office staff: ______________________

OFFICE INFO CONTINUED

Hours: ______________________

Directions: ______________________

Notes: ______________________

PATIENT PORTAL LOGIN

Website: ______________________

Login ID: ______________________

Password: ______________________

CONDITIONS MD MANAGES

____

____

____

SPECIAL INSTRUCTIONS FROM MD (WHEN TO CALL, RECOMMENDED VITAL SIGN RANGES, WHEN TO TAKE "AS NEEDED" MEDS, ETC.)

____

____

____

____

____

____

____

____

____

MD INFORMATION

MD INFO

Name: ____________________

Specialty: ____________________

Notes: ____________________

OFFICE INFO

Phone: ____________________

Address: ____________________

____

STAFF NAMES

Nurse: ____________________

PA/NP: ____________________

Office staff: ____________________

OFFICE INFO CONTINUED

Hours: ____________________

Directions: ____________________

Notes: ____________________

PATIENT PORTAL LOGIN

Website: ____________________

Login ID: ____________________

Password: ____________________

CONDITIONS MD MANAGES

____

____

____

SPECIAL INSTRUCTIONS FROM MD (WHEN TO CALL, RECOMMENDED VITAL SIGN RANGES, WHEN TO TAKE "AS NEEDED" MEDS, ETC.)

____

____

____

____

____

____

____

____

____

MD VISIT LOG

Questions to consider asking the doctor:

MEDICATIONS:

ARE THERE ANY MEDICATIONS THAT ARE NO LONGER NEEDED?

IS (CERTAIN SYMPTOM I'M HAVING) BECAUSE OF MY MEDS?

IS THERE A MEDICATION YOU RECOMMEND THAT CAN HELP WITH ______?

SHOULD ANY OF THESE MEDS BE TAKEN WITH FOOD OR ON AN EMPTY STOMACH?

SYMPTOMS:

DO YOU KNOW WHY I MIGHT BE HAVING ________ SYMPTOM?

SHOULD I BE CONCERNED ABOUT ___________ SYMPTOM?

AT WHAT POINT SHOULD I CALL SOMEONE ABOUT ________ SYMPTOM?

WOULD IT BE A GOOD IDEA TO SEE A SPECIALIST ABOUT ____ SYMPTOM?

ARE THERE ANY SUPPLEMENTS YOU RECOMMEND TO HELP WITH ______?

VITAL SIGNS:

WHAT RANGE DO YOU WANT MY (HEART RATE, BP, OXYGEN, ETC) TO STAY IN?

WHAT SHOULD I DO IF THAT VITAL SIGN IS OUTSIDE OF THAT RANGE?

DO I CALL YOU? GO TO THE EMERGENCY ROOM? TAKE A MEDICATION?

NOTE: WRITE SPECIAL RANGES IN YOUR VITAL SIGNS LOG BOOK
AND PUT DETAILED INSTRUCTIONS ON MD INFO PAGE OF THIS BOOK

FOLLOW UP:

ARE THERE ANY TESTS OR LAB WORK THAT NEEDS TO BE DONE?

IS THERE ANYTHING I NEED TO DO REGARDING MEDICATION REFILLS?

ARE THERE ANY REFERRALS TO OTHER DOCTORS THAT WILL BE MADE?

IF SO, DO I CALL THEM TO SCHEDULE OR WILL THEY CALL ME?

ANYTHING I NEED TO REPORT TO YOU BEFORE THE NEXT VISIT?

Doctor Visit

Date :

Time :

DOCTOR: ____________

OTHER: ____________

SPECIALTY: ____________

HEIGHT : ____________

NURSE: ____________

WEIGHT : ____________

CLINIC NAME: ____________

HEART RATE : ____________

LOCATION : ____________

BLOOD PRESSURE : ____________

REASON FOR VISIT

QUESTIONS I HAVE:

MD ANSWERS:

REFERRAL TO

MD NAME:

SPECIALTY:

Visit Cont.

- [ ] Does this office have the most up to date medication list?
- [ ] Do I understand how all medication from this MD should be taken?
- [ ] Am I clear about how these conditions are being handled?
- [ ] Do I understand what to do next about tests, referrals, and follow ups?
- [ ] Can I clearly explain to someone else what I learned during this visit?

MEDICATION INSTRUCTIONS

RECOMMENDATIONS/TESTS

OTHER NOTES:

FOLLOW UP ⯈ DATE : TIME :

Doctor Visit

Date :

Time :

DOCTOR: ______________________

SPECIALTY: ______________________

NURSE: ______________________

CLINIC NAME: ______________________

LOCATION : ______________________

OTHER: ______________________

HEIGHT : ______________________

WEIGHT : ______________________

HEART RATE : ______________________

BLOOD PRESSURE : ______________________

REASON FOR VISIT

QUESTIONS I HAVE:

MD ANSWERS:

REFERRAL TO

MD NAME:

SPECIALTY:

Visit Cont.

- [ ] Does this office have the most up to date medication list?
- [ ] Do I understand how all medication from this MD should be taken?
- [ ] Am I clear about how these conditions are being handled?
- [ ] Do I understand what to do next about tests, referrals, and follow ups?
- [ ] Can I clearly explain to someone else what I learned during this visit?

MEDICATION INSTRUCTIONS

RECOMMENDATIONS/TESTS

OTHER NOTES:

FOLLOW UP ▶ DATE : TIME :

Doctor Visit

Date :

Time :

DOCTOR: ______

OTHER: ______

SPECIALTY: ______

HEIGHT : ______

NURSE: ______

WEIGHT : ______

CLINIC NAME: ______

HEART RATE : ______

LOCATION : ______

BLOOD PRESSURE : ______

REASON FOR VISIT

QUESTIONS I HAVE:

MD ANSWERS:

REFERRAL TO

MD NAME:

SPECIALTY:

Visit Cont.

- [ ] Does this office have the most up to date medication list?
- [ ] Do I understand how all medication from this MD should be taken?
- [ ] Am I clear about how these conditions are being handled?
- [ ] Do I understand what to do next about tests, referrals, and follow ups?
- [ ] Can I clearly explain to someone else what I learned during this visit?

MEDICATION INSTRUCTIONS

RECOMMENDATIONS/TESTS

OTHER NOTES:

FOLLOW UP DATE : TIME :

Doctor Visit

Date :

Time :

DOCTOR: ______

OTHER: ______

SPECIALTY: ______

HEIGHT : ______

NURSE: ______

WEIGHT : ______

CLINIC NAME: ______

HEART RATE : ______

LOCATION : ______

BLOOD PRESSURE : ______

REASON FOR VISIT

QUESTIONS I HAVE:

MD ANSWERS:

REFERRAL TO

MD NAME:

SPECIALTY:

Visit Cont.

- [ ] Does this office have the most up to date medication list?
- [ ] Do I understand how all medication from this MD should be taken?
- [ ] Am I clear about how these conditions are being handled?
- [ ] Do I understand what to do next about tests, referrals, and follow ups?
- [ ] Can I clearly explain to someone else what I learned during this visit?

MEDICATION INSTRUCTIONS

RECOMMENDATIONS/TESTS

OTHER NOTES:

FOLLOW UP ⯈ DATE : TIME :

Doctor Visit

Date :

Time :

DOCTOR: ______

OTHER: ______

SPECIALTY: ______

HEIGHT : ______

NURSE: ______

WEIGHT : ______

CLINIC NAME: ______

HEART RATE : ______

LOCATION : ______

BLOOD PRESSURE : ______

REASON FOR VISIT

QUESTIONS I HAVE:

MD ANSWERS:

REFERRAL TO

MD NAME:

SPECIALTY:

Visit Cont.

- [ ] Does this office have the most up to date medication list?
- [ ] Do I understand how all medication from this MD should be taken?
- [ ] Am I clear about how these conditions are being handled?
- [ ] Do I understand what to do next about tests, referrals, and follow ups?
- [ ] Can I clearly explain to someone else what I learned during this visit?

MEDICATION INSTRUCTIONS

RECOMMENDATIONS/TESTS

OTHER NOTES:

FOLLOW UP ▶ DATE : TIME :

Doctor Visit

Date :

Time :

DOCTOR: ____________

OTHER: ____________

SPECIALTY: ____________

HEIGHT : ____________

NURSE: ____________

WEIGHT : ____________

CLINIC NAME: ____________

HEART RATE : ____________

LOCATION : ____________

BLOOD PRESSURE : ____________

REASON FOR VISIT

QUESTIONS I HAVE:

MD ANSWERS:

REFERRAL TO

MD NAME:

SPECIALTY:

Visit Cont.

- [ ] Does this office have the most up to date medication list?
- [ ] Do I understand how all medication from this MD should be taken?
- [ ] Am I clear about how these conditions are being handled?
- [ ] Do I understand what to do next about tests, referrals, and follow ups?
- [ ] Can I clearly explain to someone else what I learned during this visit?

MEDICATION INSTRUCTIONS

RECOMMENDATIONS/TESTS

OTHER NOTES:

FOLLOW UP ▶ DATE : TIME :

Doctor Visit

Date :

Time :

DOCTOR: ______

OTHER: ______

SPECIALTY: ______

HEIGHT : ______

NURSE: ______

WEIGHT : ______

CLINIC NAME: ______

HEART RATE : ______

LOCATION : ______

BLOOD PRESSURE : ______

REASON FOR VISIT

QUESTIONS I HAVE:

MD ANSWERS:

REFERRAL TO

MD NAME:

SPECIALTY:

Visit Cont.

- [ ] Does this office have the most up to date medication list?
- [ ] Do I understand how all medication from this MD should be taken?
- [ ] Am I clear about how these conditions are being handled?
- [ ] Do I understand what to do next about tests, referrals, and follow ups?
- [ ] Can I clearly explain to someone else what I learned during this visit?

MEDICATION INSTRUCTIONS

RECOMMENDATIONS/TESTS

OTHER NOTES:

FOLLOW UP ⏩ DATE : TIME :

Doctor Visit

Date :

Time :

DOCTOR: ______

OTHER: ______

SPECIALTY: ______

HEIGHT : ______

NURSE: ______

WEIGHT : ______

CLINIC NAME: ______

HEART RATE : ______

LOCATION : ______

BLOOD PRESSURE : ______

REASON FOR VISIT

QUESTIONS I HAVE:

MD ANSWERS:

REFERRAL TO

MD NAME:

SPECIALTY:

Visit Cont.

- [ ] Does this office have the most up to date medication list?
- [ ] Do I understand how all medication from this MD should be taken?
- [ ] Am I clear about how these conditions are being handled?
- [ ] Do I understand what to do next about tests, referrals, and follow ups?
- [ ] Can I clearly explain to someone else what I learned during this visit?

MEDICATION INSTRUCTIONS

RECOMMENDATIONS/TESTS

OTHER NOTES:

FOLLOW UP ⏩ DATE : TIME :

Doctor Visit

Date :

Time :

DOCTOR: ______

OTHER: ______

SPECIALTY: ______

HEIGHT : ______

NURSE: ______

WEIGHT : ______

CLINIC NAME: ______

HEART RATE : ______

LOCATION : ______

BLOOD PRESSURE : ______

REASON FOR VISIT

QUESTIONS I HAVE:

MD ANSWERS:

REFERRAL TO

MD NAME:

SPECIALTY:

Visit Cont.

- [ ] Does this office have the most up to date medication list?
- [ ] Do I understand how all medication from this MD should be taken?
- [ ] Am I clear about how these conditions are being handled?
- [ ] Do I understand what to do next about tests, referrals, and follow ups?
- [ ] Can I clearly explain to someone else what I learned during this visit?

MEDICATION INSTRUCTIONS

RECOMMENDATIONS/TESTS

OTHER NOTES:

FOLLOW UP ⯈ DATE : TIME :

Doctor Visit

Date :

Time :

DOCTOR: ______________________

OTHER: ______________________

SPECIALTY: ______________________

HEIGHT : ______________________

NURSE: ______________________

WEIGHT : ______________________

CLINIC NAME: ______________________

HEART RATE : ______________________

LOCATION : ______________________

BLOOD PRESSURE : ______________________

REASON FOR VISIT

QUESTIONS I HAVE:

MD ANSWERS:

REFERRAL TO

MD NAME:

SPECIALTY:

Visit Cont.

- [ ] Does this office have the most up to date medication list?
- [ ] Do I understand how all medication from this MD should be taken?
- [ ] Am I clear about how these conditions are being handled?
- [ ] Do I understand what to do next about tests, referrals, and follow ups?
- [ ] Can I clearly explain to someone else what I learned during this visit?

MEDICATION INSTRUCTIONS

RECOMMENDATIONS/TESTS

OTHER NOTES:

FOLLOW UP ⯈ DATE : TIME :

Doctor Visit

Date :

Time :

DOCTOR:

OTHER:

SPECIALTY:

HEIGHT :

NURSE:

WEIGHT :

CLINIC NAME:

HEART RATE :

LOCATION :

BLOOD PRESSURE :

REASON FOR VISIT

QUESTIONS I HAVE:

MD ANSWERS:

REFERRAL TO

MD NAME:

SPECIALTY:

Visit Cont.

- ☐ Does this office have the most up to date medication list?
- ☐ Do I understand how all medication from this MD should be taken?
- ☐ Am I clear about how these conditions are being handled?
- ☐ Do I understand what to do next about tests, referrals, and follow ups?
- ☐ Can I clearly explain to someone else what I learned during this visit?

MEDICATION INSTRUCTIONS

RECOMMENDATIONS/TESTS

OTHER NOTES:

FOLLOW UP ▶ DATE : TIME :

Doctor Visit

Date :

Time :

DOCTOR: ______________

OTHER: ______________

SPECIALTY: ______________

HEIGHT : ______________

NURSE: ______________

WEIGHT : ______________

CLINIC NAME: ______________

HEART RATE : ______________

LOCATION : ______________

BLOOD PRESSURE : ______________

REASON FOR VISIT

QUESTIONS I HAVE:

MD ANSWERS:

REFERRAL TO

MD NAME:

SPECIALTY:

Visit Cont.

- ☐ Does this office have the most up to date medication list?
- ☐ Do I understand how all medication from this MD should be taken?
- ☐ Am I clear about how these conditions are being handled?
- ☐ Do I understand what to do next about tests, referrals, and follow ups?
- ☐ Can I clearly explain to someone else what I learned during this visit?

MEDICATION INSTRUCTIONS

RECOMMENDATIONS/TESTS

OTHER NOTES:

FOLLOW UP ▶▶ DATE : TIME :

Doctor Visit

Date :

Time :

DOCTOR: ______________________

OTHER: ______________________

SPECIALTY: ______________________

HEIGHT : ______________________

NURSE: ______________________

WEIGHT : ______________________

CLINIC NAME: ______________________

HEART RATE : ______________________

LOCATION : ______________________

BLOOD PRESSURE : ______________________

REASON FOR VISIT

QUESTIONS I HAVE:

MD ANSWERS:

REFERRAL TO

MD NAME:

SPECIALTY:

Visit Cont.

- [ ] Does this office have the most up to date medication list?
- [ ] Do I understand how all medication from this MD should be taken?
- [ ] Am I clear about how these conditions are being handled?
- [ ] Do I understand what to do next about tests, referrals, and follow ups?
- [ ] Can I clearly explain to someone else what I learned during this visit?

MEDICATION INSTRUCTIONS

RECOMMENDATIONS/TESTS

OTHER NOTES:

FOLLOW UP ⯈ DATE : TIME :

Doctor Visit

Date :

Time :

DOCTOR:

OTHER:

SPECIALTY:

HEIGHT :

NURSE:

WEIGHT :

CLINIC NAME:

HEART RATE :

LOCATION :

BLOOD PRESSURE :

REASON FOR VISIT

QUESTIONS I HAVE:

MD ANSWERS:

REFERRAL TO

MD NAME:

SPECIALTY:

Visit Cont.

- [ ] Does this office have the most up to date medication list?
- [ ] Do I understand how all medication from this MD should be taken?
- [ ] Am I clear about how these conditions are being handled?
- [ ] Do I understand what to do next about tests, referrals, and follow ups?
- [ ] Can I clearly explain to someone else what I learned during this visit?

MEDICATION INSTRUCTIONS

RECOMMENDATIONS/TESTS

OTHER NOTES:

FOLLOW UP ⯈ DATE : TIME :

Doctor Visit

Date :

Time :

DOCTOR: ______

OTHER: ______

SPECIALTY: ______

HEIGHT : ______

NURSE: ______

WEIGHT : ______

CLINIC NAME: ______

HEART RATE : ______

LOCATION : ______

BLOOD PRESSURE : ______

REASON FOR VISIT

QUESTIONS I HAVE:

MD ANSWERS:

REFERRAL TO

MD NAME:

SPECIALTY:

Visit Cont.

- [ ] Does this office have the most up to date medication list?
- [ ] Do I understand how all medication from this MD should be taken?
- [ ] Am I clear about how these conditions are being handled?
- [ ] Do I understand what to do next about tests, referrals, and follow ups?
- [ ] Can I clearly explain to someone else what I learned during this visit?

MEDICATION INSTRUCTIONS

RECOMMENDATIONS/TESTS

OTHER NOTES:

FOLLOW UP DATE : TIME :

Doctor Visit

Date :

Time :

DOCTOR: ____________________

SPECIALTY: ____________________

NURSE: ____________________

CLINIC NAME: ____________________

LOCATION : ____________________

OTHER: ____________________

HEIGHT : ____________________

WEIGHT : ____________________

HEART RATE : ____________________

BLOOD PRESSURE : ____________________

REASON FOR VISIT

QUESTIONS I HAVE:

MD ANSWERS:

REFERRAL TO

MD NAME:

SPECIALTY:

Visit Cont.

- [ ] Does this office have the most up to date medication list?
- [ ] Do I understand how all medication from this MD should be taken?
- [ ] Am I clear about how these conditions are being handled?
- [ ] Do I understand what to do next about tests, referrals, and follow ups?
- [ ] Can I clearly explain to someone else what I learned during this visit?

MEDICATION INSTRUCTIONS

RECOMMENDATIONS/TESTS

OTHER NOTES:

FOLLOW UP ⏩ DATE : TIME :

Doctor Visit

Date :

Time :

DOCTOR: ______

OTHER: ______

SPECIALTY: ______

HEIGHT : ______

NURSE: ______

WEIGHT : ______

CLINIC NAME: ______

HEART RATE : ______

LOCATION : ______

BLOOD PRESSURE : ______

REASON FOR VISIT

QUESTIONS I HAVE:

MD ANSWERS:

REFERRAL TO

MD NAME:

SPECIALTY:

Visit Cont.

- ☐ Does this office have the most up to date medication list?
- ☐ Do I understand how all medication from this MD should be taken?
- ☐ Am I clear about how these conditions are being handled?
- ☐ Do I understand what to do next about tests, referrals, and follow ups?
- ☐ Can I clearly explain to someone else what I learned during this visit?

MEDICATION INSTRUCTIONS

RECOMMENDATIONS/TESTS

OTHER NOTES:

FOLLOW UP ▶ DATE : TIME :

Doctor Visit

Date :

Time :

DOCTOR:

OTHER:

SPECIALTY:

HEIGHT :

NURSE:

WEIGHT :

CLINIC NAME:

HEART RATE :

LOCATION :

BLOOD PRESSURE :

REASON FOR VISIT

QUESTIONS I HAVE:

MD ANSWERS:

REFERRAL TO

MD NAME:

SPECIALTY:

Visit Cont.

- [ ] Does this office have the most up to date medication list?
- [ ] Do I understand how all medication from this MD should be taken?
- [ ] Am I clear about how these conditions are being handled?
- [ ] Do I understand what to do next about tests, referrals, and follow ups?
- [ ] Can I clearly explain to someone else what I learned during this visit?

MEDICATION INSTRUCTIONS

RECOMMENDATIONS/TESTS

OTHER NOTES:

FOLLOW UP DATE : TIME :

Doctor Visit

Date :

Time :

DOCTOR: ____________

OTHER: ____________

SPECIALTY: ____________

HEIGHT : ____________

NURSE: ____________

WEIGHT : ____________

CLINIC NAME: ____________

HEART RATE : ____________

LOCATION : ____________

BLOOD PRESSURE : ____________

REASON FOR VISIT

QUESTIONS I HAVE:

MD ANSWERS:

REFERRAL TO ▶ MD NAME:

SPECIALTY:

Visit Cont.

- [ ] Does this office have the most up to date medication list?
- [ ] Do I understand how all medication from this MD should be taken?
- [ ] Am I clear about how these conditions are being handled?
- [ ] Do I understand what to do next about tests, referrals, and follow ups?
- [ ] Can I clearly explain to someone else what I learned during this visit?

MEDICATION INSTRUCTIONS

RECOMMENDATIONS/TESTS

OTHER NOTES:

FOLLOW UP DATE : TIME :

Doctor Visit

Date :

Time :

DOCTOR: ______________

OTHER: ______________

SPECIALTY: ______________

HEIGHT : ______________

NURSE: ______________

WEIGHT : ______________

CLINIC NAME: ______________

HEART RATE : ______________

LOCATION : ______________

BLOOD PRESSURE : ______________

REASON FOR VISIT

QUESTIONS I HAVE:

MD ANSWERS:

REFERRAL TO

MD NAME:

SPECIALTY:

Visit Cont.

- [ ] Does this office have the most up to date medication list?
- [ ] Do I understand how all medication from this MD should be taken?
- [ ] Am I clear about how these conditions are being handled?
- [ ] Do I understand what to do next about tests, referrals, and follow ups?
- [ ] Can I clearly explain to someone else what I learned during this visit?

MEDICATION INSTRUCTIONS

RECOMMENDATIONS/TESTS

OTHER NOTES:

FOLLOW UP ⏩ DATE : TIME :

Doctor Visit

Date :

Time :

DOCTOR: ____________________

OTHER: ____________________

SPECIALTY: ____________________

HEIGHT : ____________________

NURSE: ____________________

WEIGHT : ____________________

CLINIC NAME: ____________________

HEART RATE : ____________________

LOCATION : ____________________

BLOOD PRESSURE : ____________________

REASON FOR VISIT

QUESTIONS I HAVE:

MD ANSWERS:

REFERRAL TO

MD NAME:

SPECIALTY:

Visit Cont.

- [ ] Does this office have the most up to date medication list?
- [ ] Do I understand how all medication from this MD should be taken?
- [ ] Am I clear about how these conditions are being handled?
- [ ] Do I understand what to do next about tests, referrals, and follow ups?
- [ ] Can I clearly explain to someone else what I learned during this visit?

MEDICATION INSTRUCTIONS

RECOMMENDATIONS/TESTS

OTHER NOTES:

FOLLOW UP DATE : TIME :

Doctor Visit

Date :

Time :

DOCTOR: ______

OTHER: ______

SPECIALTY: ______

HEIGHT : ______

NURSE: ______

WEIGHT : ______

CLINIC NAME: ______

HEART RATE : ______

LOCATION : ______

BLOOD PRESSURE : ______

REASON FOR VISIT

QUESTIONS I HAVE:

MD ANSWERS:

REFERRAL TO

MD NAME:

SPECIALTY:

Visit Cont.

- [ ] Does this office have the most up to date medication list?
- [ ] Do I understand how all medication from this MD should be taken?
- [ ] Am I clear about how these conditions are being handled?
- [ ] Do I understand what to do next about tests, referrals, and follow ups?
- [ ] Can I clearly explain to someone else what I learned during this visit?

MEDICATION INSTRUCTIONS

RECOMMENDATIONS/TESTS

OTHER NOTES:

FOLLOW UP DATE : TIME :

Doctor Visit

Date :

Time :

DOCTOR: ______

OTHER: ______

SPECIALTY: ______

HEIGHT : ______

NURSE: ______

WEIGHT : ______

CLINIC NAME: ______

HEART RATE : ______

LOCATION : ______

BLOOD PRESSURE : ______

REASON FOR VISIT

QUESTIONS I HAVE:

MD ANSWERS:

REFERRAL TO

MD NAME:

SPECIALTY:

Visit Cont.

- [ ] Does this office have the most up to date medication list?
- [ ] Do I understand how all medication from this MD should be taken?
- [ ] Am I clear about how these conditions are being handled?
- [ ] Do I understand what to do next about tests, referrals, and follow ups?
- [ ] Can I clearly explain to someone else what I learned during this visit?

MEDICATION INSTRUCTIONS

RECOMMENDATIONS/TESTS

OTHER NOTES:

FOLLOW UP ▶ DATE : TIME :

Doctor Visit

Date :

Time :

DOCTOR:

OTHER:

SPECIALTY:

HEIGHT :

NURSE:

WEIGHT :

CLINIC NAME:

HEART RATE :

LOCATION :

BLOOD PRESSURE :

REASON FOR VISIT

QUESTIONS I HAVE:

MD ANSWERS:

REFERRAL TO

MD NAME:

SPECIALTY:

Visit Cont.

- [ ] Does this office have the most up to date medication list?
- [ ] Do I understand how all medication from this MD should be taken?
- [ ] Am I clear about how these conditions are being handled?
- [ ] Do I understand what to do next about tests, referrals, and follow ups?
- [ ] Can I clearly explain to someone else what I learned during this visit?

MEDICATION INSTRUCTIONS

RECOMMENDATIONS/TESTS

OTHER NOTES:

FOLLOW UP DATE : TIME :

Doctor Visit

Date :

Time :

DOCTOR: ______________________

OTHER: ______________________

SPECIALTY: ______________________

HEIGHT : ______________________

NURSE: ______________________

WEIGHT : ______________________

CLINIC NAME: ______________________

HEART RATE : ______________________

LOCATION : ______________________

BLOOD PRESSURE : ______________________

REASON FOR VISIT

QUESTIONS I HAVE:

MD ANSWERS:

REFERRAL TO

MD NAME:

SPECIALTY:

Visit Cont.

- [ ] Does this office have the most up to date medication list?
- [ ] Do I understand how all medication from this MD should be taken?
- [ ] Am I clear about how these conditions are being handled?
- [ ] Do I understand what to do next about tests, referrals, and follow ups?
- [ ] Can I clearly explain to someone else what I learned during this visit?

MEDICATION INSTRUCTIONS

RECOMMENDATIONS/TESTS

OTHER NOTES:

FOLLOW UP ⏩ DATE : TIME :

Doctor Visit

Date :

Time :

DOCTOR:

OTHER:

SPECIALTY:

HEIGHT :

NURSE:

WEIGHT :

CLINIC NAME:

HEART RATE :

LOCATION :

BLOOD PRESSURE :

REASON FOR VISIT

QUESTIONS I HAVE:

MD ANSWERS:

REFERRAL TO

MD NAME:

SPECIALTY:

Visit Cont.

- [ ] Does this office have the most up to date medication list?
- [ ] Do I understand how all medication from this MD should be taken?
- [ ] Am I clear about how these conditions are being handled?
- [ ] Do I understand what to do next about tests, referrals, and follow ups?
- [ ] Can I clearly explain to someone else what I learned during this visit?

MEDICATION INSTRUCTIONS

RECOMMENDATIONS/TESTS

OTHER NOTES:

FOLLOW UP DATE : TIME :

Doctor Visit

Date :

Time :

DOCTOR: ____________________

SPECIALTY: ____________________

NURSE: ____________________

CLINIC NAME: ____________________

LOCATION : ____________________

OTHER: ____________________

HEIGHT : ____________________

WEIGHT : ____________________

HEART RATE : ____________________

BLOOD PRESSURE : ____________________

REASON FOR VISIT

QUESTIONS I HAVE:

MD ANSWERS:

REFERRAL TO

MD NAME:

SPECIALTY:

Visit Cont.

- [ ] Does this office have the most up to date medication list?
- [ ] Do I understand how all medication from this MD should be taken?
- [ ] Am I clear about how these conditions are being handled?
- [ ] Do I understand what to do next about tests, referrals, and follow ups?
- [ ] Can I clearly explain to someone else what I learned during this visit?

MEDICATION INSTRUCTIONS

RECOMMENDATIONS/TESTS

OTHER NOTES:

FOLLOW UP DATE : TIME :

Doctor Visit

Date :

Time :

DOCTOR: ______________________

OTHER: ______________________

SPECIALTY: ______________________

HEIGHT : ______________________

NURSE: ______________________

WEIGHT : ______________________

CLINIC NAME: ______________________

HEART RATE : ______________________

LOCATION : ______________________

BLOOD PRESSURE : ______________________

REASON FOR VISIT

QUESTIONS I HAVE:

MD ANSWERS:

REFERRAL TO

MD NAME:

SPECIALTY:

Visit Cont.

- [ ] Does this office have the most up to date medication list?
- [ ] Do I understand how all medication from this MD should be taken?
- [ ] Am I clear about how these conditions are being handled?
- [ ] Do I understand what to do next about tests, referrals, and follow ups?
- [ ] Can I clearly explain to someone else what I learned during this visit?

MEDICATION INSTRUCTIONS

RECOMMENDATIONS/TESTS

OTHER NOTES:

FOLLOW UP ▶ DATE : TIME :

Doctor Visit

Date :

Time :

DOCTOR:

OTHER:

SPECIALTY:

HEIGHT :

NURSE:

WEIGHT :

CLINIC NAME:

HEART RATE :

LOCATION :

BLOOD PRESSURE :

REASON FOR VISIT

QUESTIONS I HAVE:

MD ANSWERS:

REFERRAL TO

MD NAME:

SPECIALTY:

Visit Cont.

- [ ] Does this office have the most up to date medication list?
- [ ] Do I understand how all medication from this MD should be taken?
- [ ] Am I clear about how these conditions are being handled?
- [ ] Do I understand what to do next about tests, referrals, and follow ups?
- [ ] Can I clearly explain to someone else what I learned during this visit?

MEDICATION INSTRUCTIONS

RECOMMENDATIONS/TESTS

OTHER NOTES:

FOLLOW UP ▶ DATE : TIME :

Doctor Visit

Date :

Time :

DOCTOR:

OTHER:

SPECIALTY:

HEIGHT :

NURSE:

WEIGHT :

CLINIC NAME:

HEART RATE :

LOCATION :

BLOOD PRESSURE :

REASON FOR VISIT

QUESTIONS I HAVE:

MD ANSWERS:

REFERRAL TO

MD NAME:

SPECIALTY:

Visit Cont.

- [ ] Does this office have the most up to date medication list?
- [ ] Do I understand how all medication from this MD should be taken?
- [ ] Am I clear about how these conditions are being handled?
- [ ] Do I understand what to do next about tests, referrals, and follow ups?
- [ ] Can I clearly explain to someone else what I learned during this visit?

MEDICATION INSTRUCTIONS

RECOMMENDATIONS/TESTS

OTHER NOTES:

FOLLOW UP ▶ DATE : TIME :

Doctor Visit

Date :

Time :

DOCTOR: ____________________

OTHER: ____________________

SPECIALTY: ____________________

HEIGHT : ____________________

NURSE: ____________________

WEIGHT : ____________________

CLINIC NAME: ____________________

HEART RATE : ____________________

LOCATION : ____________________

BLOOD PRESSURE : ____________________

REASON FOR VISIT

QUESTIONS I HAVE:

MD ANSWERS:

REFERRAL TO

MD NAME:

SPECIALTY:

Visit Cont.

- [ ] Does this office have the most up to date medication list?
- [ ] Do I understand how all medication from this MD should be taken?
- [ ] Am I clear about how these conditions are being handled?
- [ ] Do I understand what to do next about tests, referrals, and follow ups?
- [ ] Can I clearly explain to someone else what I learned during this visit?

MEDICATION INSTRUCTIONS

RECOMMENDATIONS/TESTS

OTHER NOTES:

FOLLOW UP DATE : TIME :

Doctor Visit

Date :

Time :

DOCTOR: ______

OTHER: ______

SPECIALTY: ______

HEIGHT : ______

NURSE: ______

WEIGHT : ______

CLINIC NAME: ______

HEART RATE : ______

LOCATION : ______

BLOOD PRESSURE : ______

REASON FOR VISIT

QUESTIONS I HAVE:

MD ANSWERS:

REFERRAL TO

MD NAME:

SPECIALTY:

Visit Cont.

- [ ] Does this office have the most up to date medication list?
- [ ] Do I understand how all medication from this MD should be taken?
- [ ] Am I clear about how these conditions are being handled?
- [ ] Do I understand what to do next about tests, referrals, and follow ups?
- [ ] Can I clearly explain to someone else what I learned during this visit?

MEDICATION INSTRUCTIONS

RECOMMENDATIONS/TESTS

OTHER NOTES:

FOLLOW UP ⏩ DATE : TIME :

Doctor Visit

Date :

Time :

DOCTOR:

OTHER:

SPECIALTY:

HEIGHT :

NURSE:

WEIGHT :

CLINIC NAME:

HEART RATE :

LOCATION :

BLOOD PRESSURE :

REASON FOR VISIT

QUESTIONS I HAVE:

MD ANSWERS:

REFERRAL TO

MD NAME:

SPECIALTY:

Visit Cont.

- [ ] Does this office have the most up to date medication list?
- [ ] Do I understand how all medication from this MD should be taken?
- [ ] Am I clear about how these conditions are being handled?
- [ ] Do I understand what to do next about tests, referrals, and follow ups?
- [ ] Can I clearly explain to someone else what I learned during this visit?

MEDICATION INSTRUCTIONS

RECOMMENDATIONS/TESTS

OTHER NOTES:

FOLLOW UP ⏩ DATE : TIME :

Doctor Visit

Date :

Time :

DOCTOR: ____________________

OTHER: ____________________

SPECIALTY: ____________________

HEIGHT : ____________________

NURSE: ____________________

WEIGHT : ____________________

CLINIC NAME: ____________________

HEART RATE : ____________________

LOCATION : ____________________

BLOOD PRESSURE : ____________________

REASON FOR VISIT

QUESTIONS I HAVE:

MD ANSWERS:

REFERRAL TO

MD NAME:

SPECIALTY:

Visit Cont.

- [ ] Does this office have the most up to date medication list?
- [ ] Do I understand how all medication from this MD should be taken?
- [ ] Am I clear about how these conditions are being handled?
- [ ] Do I understand what to do next about tests, referrals, and follow ups?
- [ ] Can I clearly explain to someone else what I learned during this visit?

MEDICATION INSTRUCTIONS

RECOMMENDATIONS/TESTS

OTHER NOTES:

FOLLOW UP ⯈ DATE : TIME :

Doctor Visit

Date :

Time :

DOCTOR: ______________________

OTHER: ______________________

SPECIALTY: ______________________

HEIGHT : ______________________

NURSE: ______________________

WEIGHT : ______________________

CLINIC NAME: ______________________

HEART RATE : ______________________

LOCATION : ______________________

BLOOD PRESSURE : ______________________

REASON FOR VISIT

QUESTIONS I HAVE:

MD ANSWERS:

REFERRAL TO

MD NAME:

SPECIALTY:

Visit Cont.

- [ ] Does this office have the most up to date medication list?
- [ ] Do I understand how all medication from this MD should be taken?
- [ ] Am I clear about how these conditions are being handled?
- [ ] Do I understand what to do next about tests, referrals, and follow ups?
- [ ] Can I clearly explain to someone else what I learned during this visit?

MEDICATION INSTRUCTIONS

RECOMMENDATIONS/TESTS

OTHER NOTES:

FOLLOW UP ⏩ DATE : TIME :

Doctor Visit

Date :

Time :

DOCTOR:	OTHER:
SPECIALTY:	HEIGHT :
NURSE:	WEIGHT :
CLINIC NAME:	HEART RATE :
LOCATION :	BLOOD PRESSURE :

REASON FOR VISIT

QUESTIONS I HAVE:

MD ANSWERS:

REFERRAL TO ▶ MD NAME: SPECIALTY:

Visit Cont.

- [ ] Does this office have the most up to date medication list?
- [ ] Do I understand how all medication from this MD should be taken?
- [ ] Am I clear about how these conditions are being handled?
- [ ] Do I understand what to do next about tests, referrals, and follow ups?
- [ ] Can I clearly explain to someone else what I learned during this visit?

MEDICATION INSTRUCTIONS

RECOMMENDATIONS/TESTS

OTHER NOTES:

FOLLOW UP ▶ DATE : TIME :

Doctor Visit

Date :

Time :

DOCTOR: ______________________

OTHER: ______________________

SPECIALTY: ______________________

HEIGHT : ______________________

NURSE: ______________________

WEIGHT : ______________________

CLINIC NAME: ______________________

HEART RATE : ______________________

LOCATION : ______________________

BLOOD PRESSURE : ______________________

REASON FOR VISIT

QUESTIONS I HAVE:

MD ANSWERS:

REFERRAL TO

MD NAME:

SPECIALTY:

Visit Cont.

- [ ] Does this office have the most up to date medication list?
- [ ] Do I understand how all medication from this MD should be taken?
- [ ] Am I clear about how these conditions are being handled?
- [ ] Do I understand what to do next about tests, referrals, and follow ups?
- [ ] Can I clearly explain to someone else what I learned during this visit?

MEDICATION INSTRUCTIONS

RECOMMENDATIONS/TESTS

OTHER NOTES:

FOLLOW UP ⏩ DATE : TIME :

Doctor Visit

Date :

Time :

DOCTOR:

OTHER:

SPECIALTY:

HEIGHT :

NURSE:

WEIGHT :

CLINIC NAME:

HEART RATE :

LOCATION :

BLOOD PRESSURE :

REASON FOR VISIT

QUESTIONS I HAVE:

MD ANSWERS:

REFERRAL TO

MD NAME:

SPECIALTY:

Visit Cont.

- [ ] Does this office have the most up to date medication list?
- [ ] Do I understand how all medication from this MD should be taken?
- [ ] Am I clear about how these conditions are being handled?
- [ ] Do I understand what to do next about tests, referrals, and follow ups?
- [ ] Can I clearly explain to someone else what I learned during this visit?

MEDICATION INSTRUCTIONS

RECOMMENDATIONS/TESTS

OTHER NOTES:

FOLLOW UP ▶ DATE : TIME :

Doctor Visit

Date :

Time :

DOCTOR: ______

OTHER: ______

SPECIALTY: ______

HEIGHT : ______

NURSE: ______

WEIGHT : ______

CLINIC NAME: ______

HEART RATE : ______

LOCATION : ______

BLOOD PRESSURE : ______

REASON FOR VISIT

QUESTIONS I HAVE:

MD ANSWERS:

REFERRAL TO

MD NAME:

SPECIALTY:

Visit Cont.

- [ ] Does this office have the most up to date medication list?
- [ ] Do I understand how all medication from this MD should be taken?
- [ ] Am I clear about how these conditions are being handled?
- [ ] Do I understand what to do next about tests, referrals, and follow ups?
- [ ] Can I clearly explain to someone else what I learned during this visit?

MEDICATION INSTRUCTIONS

RECOMMENDATIONS/TESTS

OTHER NOTES:

FOLLOW UP ⯈ DATE : TIME :

Doctor Visit

Date :

Time :

DOCTOR: ______

OTHER: ______

SPECIALTY: ______

HEIGHT : ______

NURSE: ______

WEIGHT : ______

CLINIC NAME: ______

HEART RATE : ______

LOCATION : ______

BLOOD PRESSURE : ______

REASON FOR VISIT

QUESTIONS I HAVE:

MD ANSWERS:

REFERRAL TO

MD NAME:

SPECIALTY:

Visit Cont.

- [ ] Does this office have the most up to date medication list?
- [ ] Do I understand how all medication from this MD should be taken?
- [ ] Am I clear about how these conditions are being handled?
- [ ] Do I understand what to do next about tests, referrals, and follow ups?
- [ ] Can I clearly explain to someone else what I learned during this visit?

MEDICATION INSTRUCTIONS

RECOMMENDATIONS/TESTS

OTHER NOTES:

FOLLOW UP ⯈ DATE : TIME :

Doctor Visit

Date :

Time :

DOCTOR: ______

OTHER: ______

SPECIALTY: ______

HEIGHT : ______

NURSE: ______

WEIGHT : ______

CLINIC NAME: ______

HEART RATE : ______

LOCATION : ______

BLOOD PRESSURE : ______

REASON FOR VISIT

QUESTIONS I HAVE:

MD ANSWERS:

REFERRAL TO

MD NAME:

SPECIALTY:

Visit Cont.

- [ ] Does this office have the most up to date medication list?
- [ ] Do I understand how all medication from this MD should be taken?
- [ ] Am I clear about how these conditions are being handled?
- [ ] Do I understand what to do next about tests, referrals, and follow ups?
- [ ] Can I clearly explain to someone else what I learned during this visit?

MEDICATION INSTRUCTIONS

RECOMMENDATIONS/TESTS

OTHER NOTES:

FOLLOW UP DATE : TIME :

Doctor Visit

Date :

Time :

DOCTOR: ______________________

OTHER: ______________________

SPECIALTY: ______________________

HEIGHT : ______________________

NURSE: ______________________

WEIGHT : ______________________

CLINIC NAME: ______________________

HEART RATE : ______________________

LOCATION : ______________________

BLOOD PRESSURE : ______________________

REASON FOR VISIT

QUESTIONS I HAVE:

MD ANSWERS:

REFERRAL TO

MD NAME:

SPECIALTY:

Visit Cont.

- [ ] Does this office have the most up to date medication list?
- [ ] Do I understand how all medication from this MD should be taken?
- [ ] Am I clear about how these conditions are being handled?
- [ ] Do I understand what to do next about tests, referrals, and follow ups?
- [ ] Can I clearly explain to someone else what I learned during this visit?

MEDICATION INSTRUCTIONS

RECOMMENDATIONS/TESTS

OTHER NOTES:

FOLLOW UP ⯈ DATE : TIME :

Doctor Visit

Date :

Time :

DOCTOR:

OTHER:

SPECIALTY:

HEIGHT :

NURSE:

WEIGHT :

CLINIC NAME:

HEART RATE :

LOCATION :

BLOOD PRESSURE :

REASON FOR VISIT

QUESTIONS I HAVE:

MD ANSWERS:

REFERRAL TO

MD NAME:

SPECIALTY:

Visit Cont.

- [ ] Does this office have the most up to date medication list?
- [ ] Do I understand how all medication from this MD should be taken?
- [ ] Am I clear about how these conditions are being handled?
- [ ] Do I understand what to do next about tests, referrals, and follow ups?
- [ ] Can I clearly explain to someone else what I learned during this visit?

MEDICATION INSTRUCTIONS

RECOMMENDATIONS/TESTS

OTHER NOTES:

FOLLOW UP DATE : TIME :

Doctor Visit

Date :

Time :

DOCTOR:

OTHER:

SPECIALTY:

HEIGHT :

NURSE:

WEIGHT :

CLINIC NAME:

HEART RATE :

LOCATION :

BLOOD PRESSURE :

REASON FOR VISIT

QUESTIONS I HAVE:

MD ANSWERS:

REFERRAL TO

MD NAME:

SPECIALTY:

Visit Cont.

- [ ] Does this office have the most up to date medication list?
- [ ] Do I understand how all medication from this MD should be taken?
- [ ] Am I clear about how these conditions are being handled?
- [ ] Do I understand what to do next about tests, referrals, and follow ups?
- [ ] Can I clearly explain to someone else what I learned during this visit?

MEDICATION INSTRUCTIONS

RECOMMENDATIONS/TESTS

OTHER NOTES:

FOLLOW UP ⏩ DATE : TIME :

Doctor Visit

Date :

Time :

DOCTOR: ____________________

OTHER: ____________________

SPECIALTY: ____________________

HEIGHT : ____________________

NURSE: ____________________

WEIGHT : ____________________

CLINIC NAME: ____________________

HEART RATE : ____________________

LOCATION : ____________________

BLOOD PRESSURE : ____________________

REASON FOR VISIT

QUESTIONS I HAVE:

MD ANSWERS:

REFERRAL TO

MD NAME:

SPECIALTY:

Visit Cont.

- [ ] Does this office have the most up to date medication list?
- [ ] Do I understand how all medication from this MD should be taken?
- [ ] Am I clear about how these conditions are being handled?
- [ ] Do I understand what to do next about tests, referrals, and follow ups?
- [ ] Can I clearly explain to someone else what I learned during this visit?

MEDICATION INSTRUCTIONS

RECOMMENDATIONS/TESTS

OTHER NOTES:

FOLLOW UP ⮞ DATE : TIME :

Doctor Visit

Date :

Time :

DOCTOR:

SPECIALTY:

NURSE:

CLINIC NAME:

LOCATION :

OTHER:

HEIGHT :

WEIGHT :

HEART RATE :

BLOOD PRESSURE :

REASON FOR VISIT

QUESTIONS I HAVE:

MD ANSWERS:

REFERRAL TO

MD NAME:

SPECIALTY:

Visit Cont.

- [ ] Does this office have the most up to date medication list?
- [ ] Do I understand how all medication from this MD should be taken?
- [ ] Am I clear about how these conditions are being handled?
- [ ] Do I understand what to do next about tests, referrals, and follow ups?
- [ ] Can I clearly explain to someone else what I learned during this visit?

MEDICATION INSTRUCTIONS

RECOMMENDATIONS/TESTS

OTHER NOTES:

FOLLOW UP DATE : TIME :

Doctor Visit

Date :

Time :

DOCTOR: ____________

OTHER: ____________

SPECIALTY: ____________

HEIGHT : ____________

NURSE: ____________

WEIGHT : ____________

CLINIC NAME: ____________

HEART RATE : ____________

LOCATION : ____________

BLOOD PRESSURE : ____________

REASON FOR VISIT

QUESTIONS I HAVE:

MD ANSWERS:

REFERRAL TO

MD NAME:

SPECIALTY:

Visit Cont.

- [ ] Does this office have the most up to date medication list?
- [ ] Do I understand how all medication from this MD should be taken?
- [ ] Am I clear about how these conditions are being handled?
- [ ] Do I understand what to do next about tests, referrals, and follow ups?
- [ ] Can I clearly explain to someone else what I learned during this visit?

MEDICATION INSTRUCTIONS

RECOMMENDATIONS/TESTS

OTHER NOTES:

FOLLOW UP ⯈ DATE : TIME :

Doctor Visit

Date :

Time :

DOCTOR: ______________________

OTHER: ______________________

SPECIALTY: ______________________

HEIGHT : ______________________

NURSE: ______________________

WEIGHT : ______________________

CLINIC NAME: ______________________

HEART RATE : ______________________

LOCATION : ______________________

BLOOD PRESSURE : ______________________

REASON FOR VISIT

QUESTIONS I HAVE:

MD ANSWERS:

REFERRAL TO ▶ MD NAME: SPECIALTY:

Visit Cont.

- [ ] Does this office have the most up to date medication list?
- [ ] Do I understand how all medication from this MD should be taken?
- [ ] Am I clear about how these conditions are being handled?
- [ ] Do I understand what to do next about tests, referrals, and follow ups?
- [ ] Can I clearly explain to someone else what I learned during this visit?

MEDICATION INSTRUCTIONS

RECOMMENDATIONS/TESTS

OTHER NOTES:

FOLLOW UP DATE : TIME :

TESTING/SCANS/LABS

TESTING/SCANS/LABS

Date of Test	Ordered by (MD)	Reason for Test	Results/Notes:

TESTING/SCANS/LABS

Date of Test	Ordered by (MD)	Reason for Test	Results/Notes:

TESTING/SCANS/LABS

Date of Test	Ordered by (MD)	Reason for Test	Results/Notes:

TESTING/SCANS/LABS

Date of Test	Ordered by (MD)	Reason for Test	Results/Notes:

TESTING/SCANS/LABS

Date of Test	Ordered by (MD)	Reason for Test	Results/Notes:

OFFICE CALL LOG

OFFICE CALL LOG

Date of Call	Doctor's Office Called	Reason for Call	Notes from nurse/MD:

OFFICE CALL LOG

Date of Call	Doctor's Office Called	Reason for Call	Notes from nurse/MD:

OFFICE CALL LOG

Date of Call	Doctor's Office Called	Reason for Call	Notes from nurse/MD:

OFFICE CALL LOG

Date of Call	Doctor's Office Called	Reason for Call	Notes from nurse/MD:

OFFICE CALL LOG

Date of Call	Doctor's Office Called	Reason for Call	Notes from nurse/MD:

OFFICE CALL LOG

Date of Call	Doctor's Office Called	Reason for Call	Notes from nurse/MD:

OFFICE CALL LOG

Date of Call	Doctor's Office Called	Reason for Call	Notes from nurse/MD:

OFFICE CALL LOG

Date of Call	Doctor's Office Called	Reason for Call	Notes from nurse/MD:

OFFICE CALL LOG

Date of Call	Doctor's Office Called	Reason for Call	Notes from nurse/MD:

PATIENT MEDICAL HISTORY

ALLERGIES/SURGERIES

ALLERGIES:

MEDICATIONS: Always keep an up to date list in your wallet or purse. Download your FREE medication list template (that can be edited digitally and printed!) at helpthecaregiver.com/medication-list

SURGERIES:

Type of Surgery	Name of Surgeon	Date of Surgery	Notes (complications, hospital stay after and dates, etc):

SURGERIES

SURGERIES CONT:

Type of Surgery	Name of Surgeon	Date of Surgery	Notes (complications, hospital stay after and dates, etc):

HOSPITALIZATIONS

HOSPITALIZATIONS:

Date(s) of Stay	Reason for Stay	Name of Hospital	Notes (complications, tests run, new diagnosis, etc):

HOSPITALIZATIONS

HOSPITALIZATIONS CONTINUED:

Date(s) of Stay	Reason for Stay	Name of Hospital	Notes (complications, tests run, new diagnosis, etc):

HOSPITALIZATIONS

HOSPITALIZATIONS CONTINUED:

Date(s) of Stay	Reason for Stay	Name of Hospital	Notes (complications, tests run, new diagnosis, etc):

HOSPITALIZATIONS

HOSPITALIZATIONS CONTINUED:

Date(s) of Stay	Reason for Stay	Name of Hospital	Notes (complications, tests run, new diagnosis, etc):

FALLS

FALLS:

Date of Fall	Symptoms with the fall	Location of the fall	Notes (injuries, scans, MD visits, identified cause of fall, etc):

FALLS

FALLS CONTINUED:

Date of Fall	Symptoms with the fall	Location of the fall	Notes (injuries, scans, MD visits, identified cause of fall, etc):

FALLS

FALLS CONTINUED:

Date of Fall	Symptoms with the fall	Location of the fall	Notes (injuries, scans, MD visits, identified cause of fall, etc):

FALLS

FALLS CONTINUED:

Date of Fall	Symptoms with the fall	Location of the fall	Notes (injuries, scans, MD visits, identified cause of fall, etc):

ABOUT

DR. JULIE CRENSHAW

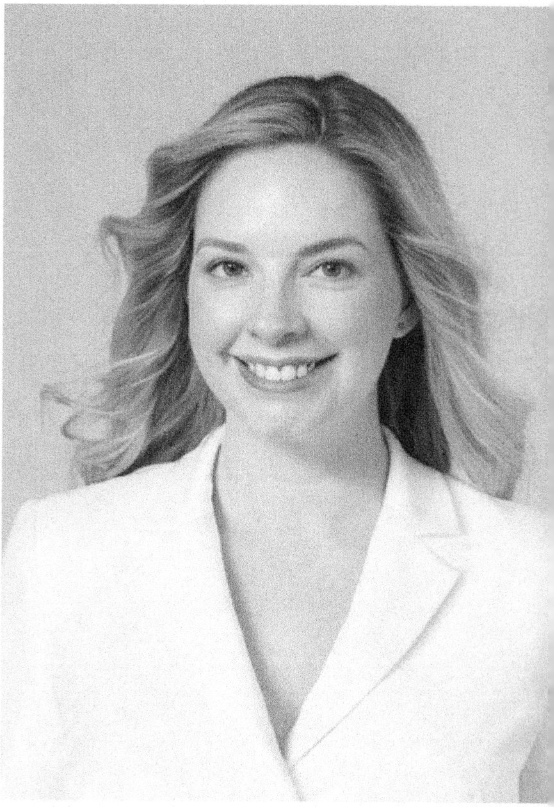

Julie started college as a music performance major playing the french horn, but ultimately pursued becoming a physical therapist to be able to give hands-on care to others. It didn't take long after graduating PT school for Julie to realize the passion she felt for working with the aging population.

It was her many years of working in home health that inspired her to found Help the Caregiver in order to create change for caregivers who she saw doing so much with so little help.

Julie was born and raised in Georgia, where she currently lives with her husband and 3 children.

She loves spending quality time with her family any way that will put her near water, whether it's by the beach, lake, pool, or hiking to a beautiful waterfall.

Books in this Series

Learn to Care for Aging Parents

The "Learn to Care for Aging Parents" series is designed for caregivers in order to empower them with knowledge and decrease overwhelm related to caring for aging loved ones.

This set of 3 books makes the perfect resource for new and long-term caregivers alike, helping to give structure and organization to caregiving needs.

Use the vital signs and MD communication log books to track important measures and keep medical information well organized. Practical tips, checklists, and troubleshooting guides available in the "Bringing a Parent Home from the Hospital" resource book give important information that can be referred to again and again.

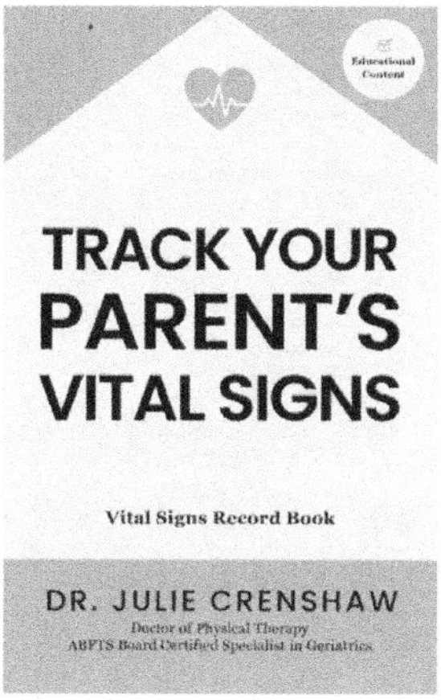

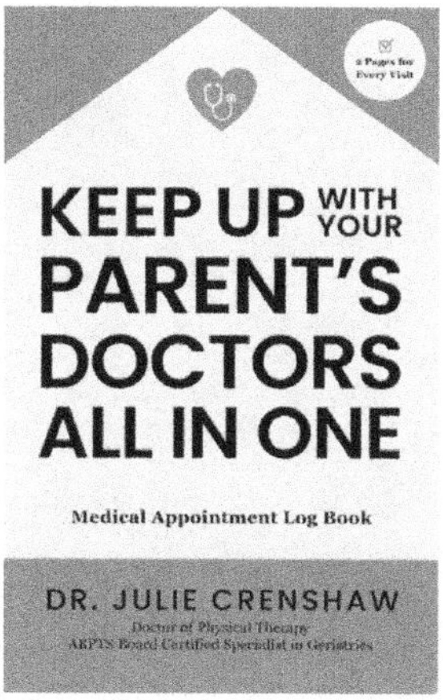

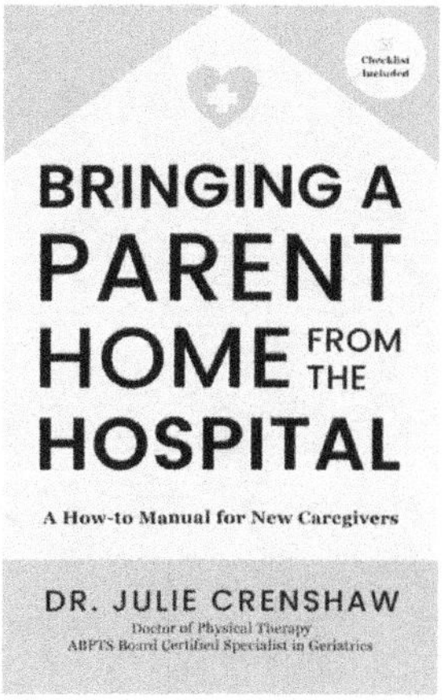

Made in the USA
Monee, IL
04 November 2026

67380084R00085